10 Minute Stretch

Written

by

Certified

Personal Fitness Trainer
and
Nutritional Specialist

Larry Holden

To order additional copies of this book, contact:
Xlibris Corporation
1-888-795-4274
www.Xlibris.com
Orders@Xlibris.com
70129

CONTENTS

Acknowledgement 5

Foreword 7

Stretching 101 11

Active Stretch 17

Stretching Techniques 23

Acknowledgement

I acknowledge with warmth and thankfulness, all my friends that help make this book possible. I salute you, and I'm honored, to count you as friends.

I'm also appreciative, of Natalie K. Holden, my wife for her suggestions throughout the writing of the manuscript.

Foreword

I've thought about writing Ten Minute Stretch for several years. I've worked side-by-side with fitness trainers, and know the importance of a stretching routine that must be part of any exercise program. My book Ten Minute Stretch is a reference book for beginner that explains the benefits it provides to people with sedentary lifestyles. As I wrote this book it became more apparent to me that it could help not only beginners, those afraid of hurting themselves, but trained athletes as well. I gathered my notes, comparisons, tips, and guidelines and put them into this specific manual.

This book is full of examples, and terms, with key informational guidelines that will be helpful not only for people new to exercising, but also those experienced. I tried to arrange the information in the most practical order, some parts of the chapters may appear to be repetitious, but that's intentional. I know you will understand the concepts better that way; I have included as many procedures with collaborative exercises that are helpful. This book has two purposes: First, to serve as a text for the role stretching can provide to people beginning an exercise program, and second, to those that are experience exercisers. My book Ten Minute Stretch is a point of reference to stretching, so stretch your way to Wellness.

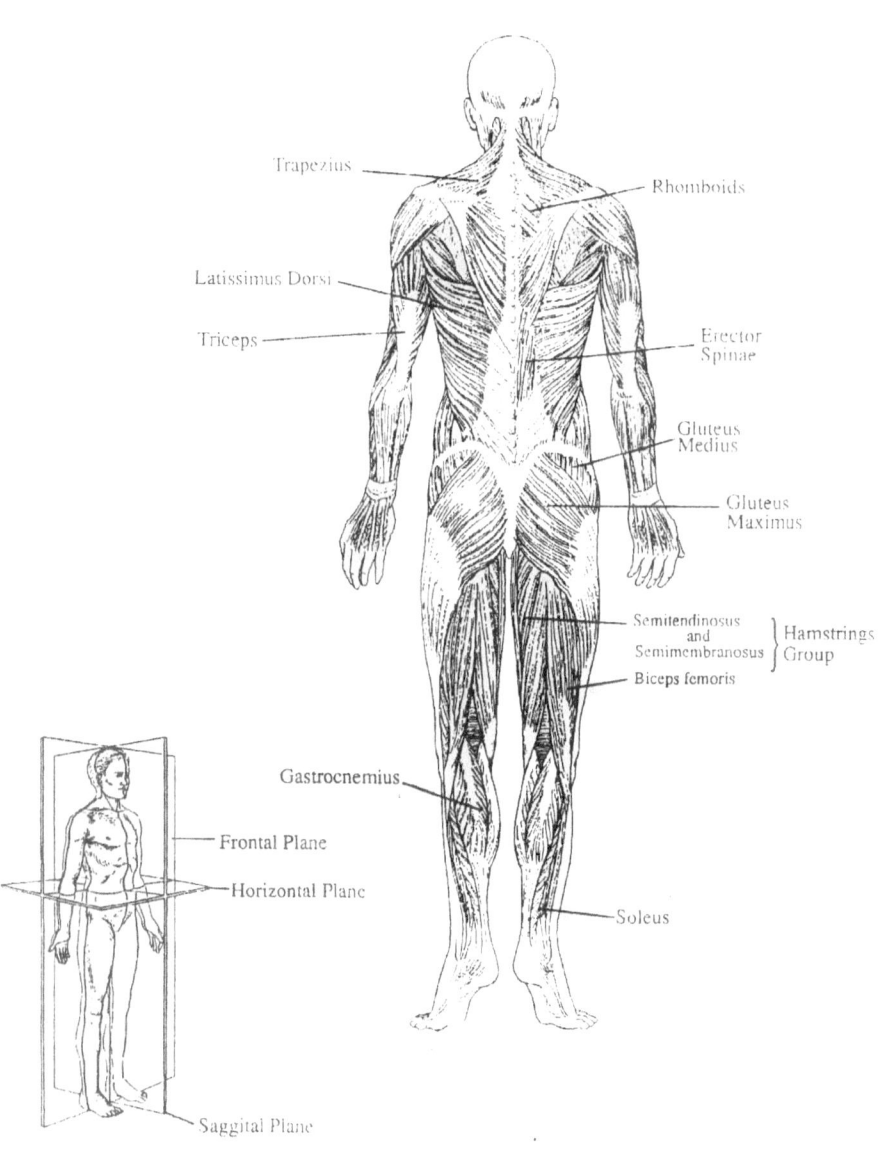

Trapezius

Rhomboids

Latissimus Dorsi

Triceps

Erector
Spinae

Gluteus
Medius

Gluteus
Maximus

Semitendinosus
and
Semimembranosus

Hamstrings
Group

Biceps femoris

Gastrocnemius

Frontal Plane

Horizontal Plane

Soleus

Saggital Plane

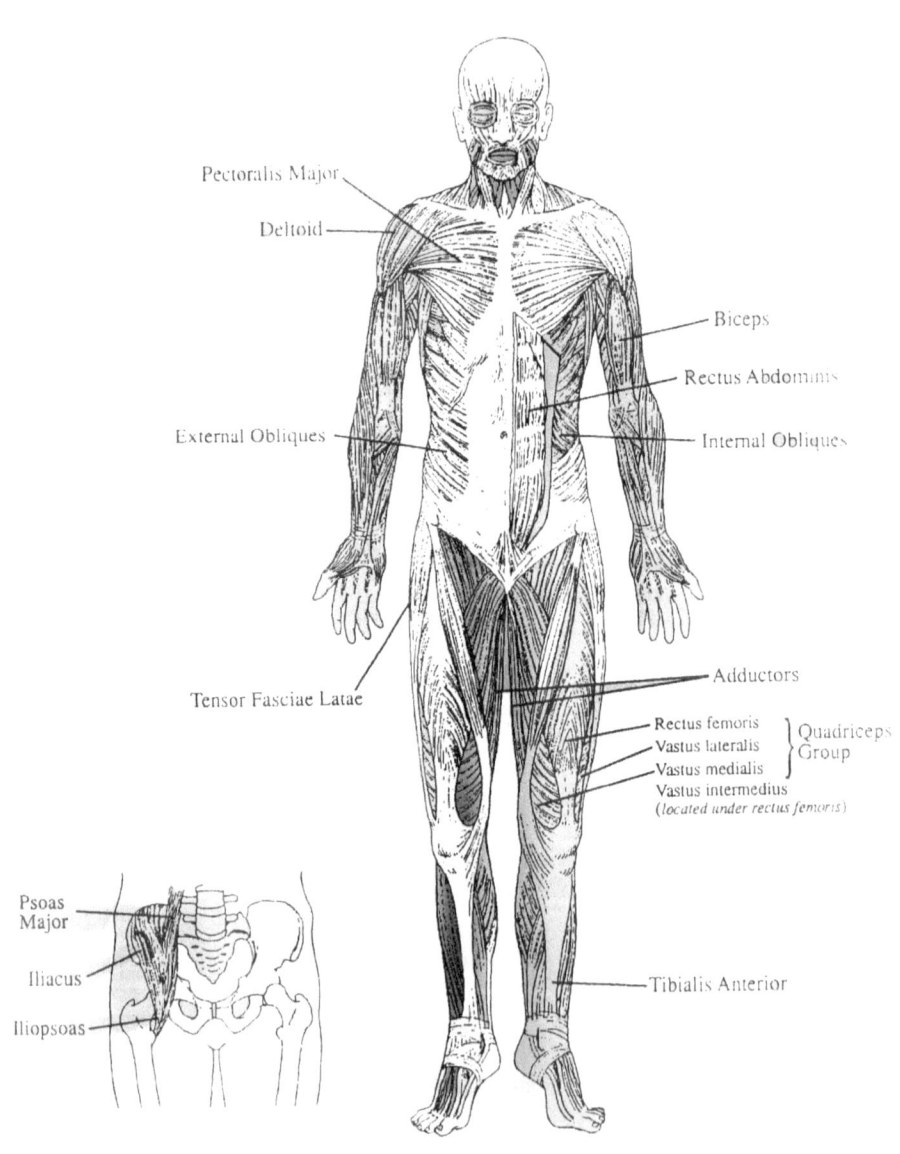

Pectoralis Major

Deltoid

Biceps

Rectus Abdominis

External Obliques

Internal Obliques

Adductors

Tensor Fasciae Latae

Rectus femoris
Vastus lateralis
Vastus medialis
Vastus intermedius
(*located under rectus femoris*)

} Quadriceps
  Group

Psoas
Major

Iliacus

Iliopsoas

Tibialis Anterior

STRETCHING 101

Basic

"Flexibility": the ability of a joint to move through its range of motion.

A full-body flexibility program will help you reduce fatigue and avoid injury when you're short on time. Proper stretching should be the first thing done. The Ten-minute stretch will get you motivated for the day with a spring in your step. As with any fitness program, first check with your physician and get medical clearance before you get involved in any training program. Cardiovascular training helps us lose weight and get fit. Strength training helps us build muscles and shed fat. Ten minute stretch done regularly will reduce fatigue and will help you avoid soft tissue injuries. The Ten Minute Stretch will increase your flexibility and help you stay limber, giving you greater functional movement of your body. You will suffer less from lower back pain and muscle strain have fewer injuries with an improved range of motion. If you want to improve your golf swing or tennis game, start with flexibility warm-ups. With ten-minute stretch, I can show you how easy and fun stretching can become as a regular part of your daily life—. Are you ready for better body tone and greater movement that will help you stay limber? These stretches done twice a day will decrease injuries and improve your overall flexibility and vitality. Are you ready? I think you are! So let's get started on ten minutes to a better life.

Benefits of Flexibility and Stretching Exercise

The prevention of lower back pain, the maintenance of good posture. The prevention and rehabilitation of muscle injuries. Reduces post exercise muscle soreness, stress management, and relaxation. Stretching will relieve pain and aches from prolonged sitting, lying, or standing positions.

Benefits of Flexibility and Stretching:

1. Prevent lower back pain.
2. Reduces post exercise muscle soreness
3. Reduces stress and promotes relaxation
4. Help ease the rehabilitation process from muscle injuries.

Along with the practice of good posture, stretching will relieve pain and aches from prolonged siting, lying, or standing poitions.

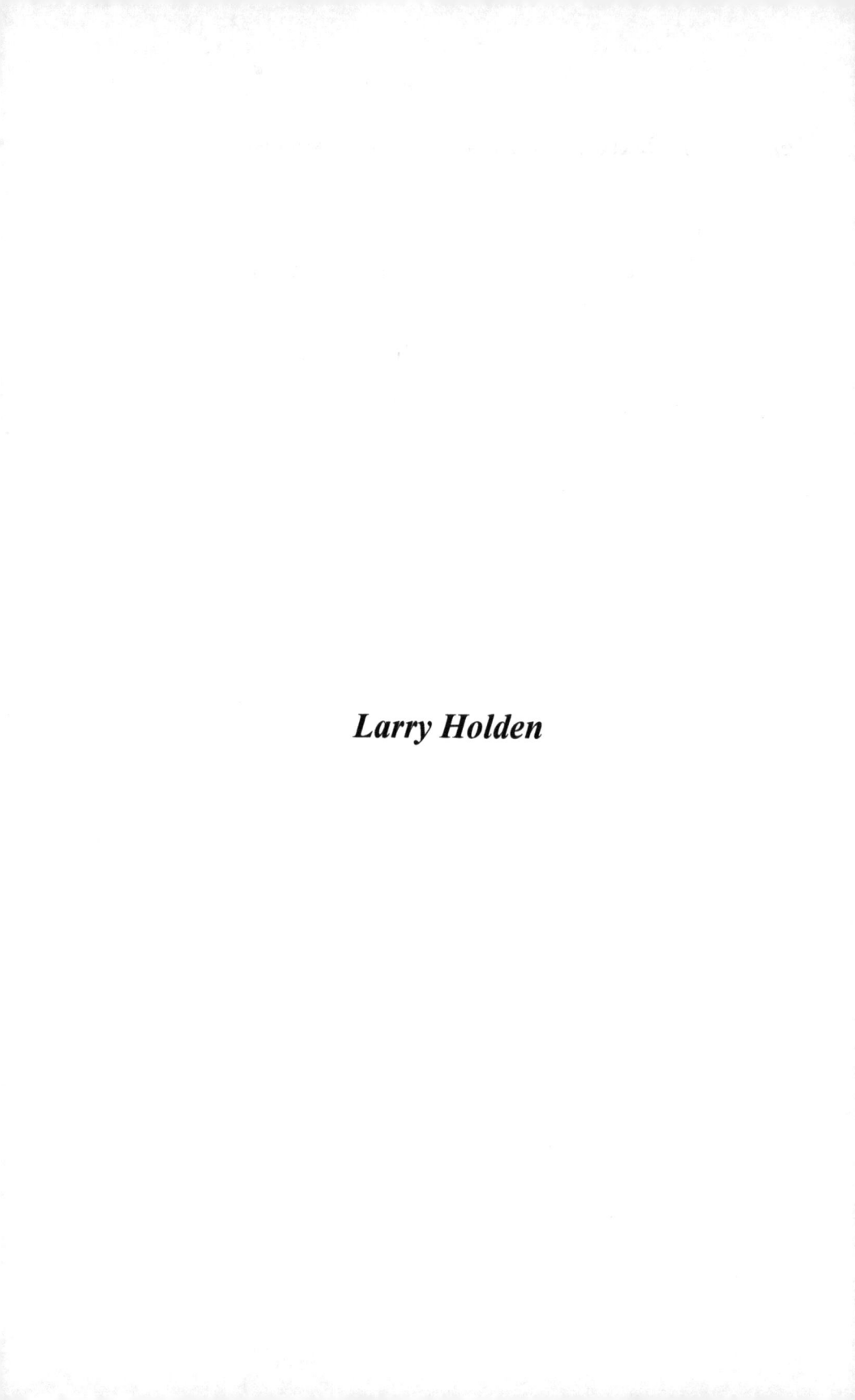

Larry Holden

ACTIVE STRETCH

Exercise Prescription:

The Goal:
To maintain adequate range of motion in daily activities

The Frequency:
Everyday, each time before and after exercise

The Intensity:
Until you feel mild discomfort in the stretch

The Time:
Hold for fifteen seconds, with repetitions of 1-3 reps, for each muscle group. Fifteen seconds can be too long, for beginners in these cases, hold as long as possible, to improve your flexibility.

Stretching Exercises

Neck: flexion, side bending, extension, rotation (head turns and tilts)

Shoulders: rotator cuff, deltoid extension, towel stretch

Front Arm: biceps stretch, arm extension, wrist extension

Back Arm: triceps stretch, arm overhead stretch

Upper Back: trapezius stretch, lateral bend, prayer stretch, chin-to-chest stretch, rotations

Lower Back: knee-to-chest stretch, trunk twist, press-up, cat-and-camel stretch, hamstring stretch

Buttocks: gluteus stretch, knee to chest, hamstring stretch, hip rotations

Outer Thigh/Hip Oblique: oblique external and internal rotation side to side, bend-over-body stretch, trunk rotation

Front Leg/Hip: standing lunge, side lunge, quadriceps stretch, sole stretch

Front Leg: standing lunge, side lunge, quadriceps stretch, sole stretch

Back Leg: hamstring stretch (standing, lying, seated) modified hurdler stretch

Inner Thigh: modified hurdler stretch, sole stretch, side lunges, adductions

Lower Leg: calf/achilles and soleus stretch, ankle plantar, dorsiflexion, ankle inversion and eversion, toe extension

Hamstrings:

Lie on your back on a mat with your left leg extended on the floor. Place a band or towel under the right foot and extend it toward the ceiling, grasping the end of the towel or band in the right hand. Now relax the quadriceps of the right leg, supporting the weight of this leg with the band or towel and your right arm until you feel slight discomfort. Hold this position about 15-30 seconds as you slowly and evenly breathe. If the stretch is effortlessness, use your right arm or band to pull the leg closer toward your face to the point where you have a deep stretch and the pelvic has not moved. Repeat this stretch with the other leg. Two to three repetitions, three sets.

Quadriceps Stretch: Stand and support yourself against a wall with one hand, keeping your abs engaged as you slowly and evenly breathe. Lift one leg up and bend it back, holding it in place with your hand until you feel a stretch for about 15-30 seconds. Repeat this stretch with the other leg 2-3 repetitions, 3 sets.

Triceps Stretch: Sit on a fitball or chair without a backrest. Keeping your abs engaged, hold a band or a large drying towel in both hands place them behind your back. With both arms behind your back, pull the upper arm down toward the lower back using the band or large drying towel until you feel a stretch. Repeat this stretch with the other arm 5-10 seconds. Each arm, 5-10 repetitions, 3 sets.

Shoulder-over-Bridge Stretch: Measures the flexibility of shoulder joint, deltoids, and pectoralis major.

Sit on a fitball or chair without backrest, keeping your abs engaged as you slowly and evenly breathe. Bring your right arm over your head down the center of the back, with your fingertips touching the middle area of your spine. With your other arm reaching up from the center as far as you can, reach hold for 5-10 seconds. Repeat this stretch with the other arm, 5-10 repetitions 3 sets. Take a deep breath and remember to stretch only until you feel slight discomfort in each muscle group you are working. The diagram of the human muscular system will help you to identify each muscle group and their locations, showing all the parts of that system. Study them, and stretch them.

STRETCHING TECHNIQUES

Static Stretching: A technique in which a muscle is slowly and gently stretched and then held in the stretched position for 30-60 seconds.

Recommended technique: Passive stretching versus active stretching

Ballistic Stretching: A technique in which muscles are stretched by force generated as a body part is repeatedly bounced, swung, or jerked. Due to the stimulation of the stretch reflex, this type of stretching is not recommended.

Proprioceptive Neuromuscular Facilitation (PNF)

A technique in which an inverse stretch reflex induces relaxation in a muscle prior to it being stretched, allowing for more stretch and more rapid development of joint flexibility. This technique is not for beginners, but is very effective. When stretching the hamstring, your partner pushes the hamstring (antagonist) toward your chest while you push your thigh against the partner who is pressing your leg towards you. Hold the stretch for 5-6 seconds by pushing your leg toward chest of your partner. The muscle group is then relaxed and a controlled stretch is applied for about 20 to 30 seconds. The muscle group is then allowed 30 seconds to recover and the process is repeated 2-4 times.

Neck: Flexion, Side Bending, Extension, Rotation Head Turns And Tilts

Neck Extension: Slowly tilt your head back and look up at the ceiling. Place one hand on your forehead to gently assist this motion. Stop when a stretch is felt in the muscles in the front of your neck. Hold for a count of ten.

Neck Rotation: Slowly turn your head and look over your left shoulder. Place one hand on your right check to gently assist this motion. Stop when a stretch is felt in the muscles on the right side of your neck. Hold for a count of ten. Repeat the steps above in the opposite direction

Side Flexion: Slowly tilt your left ear down to your left shoulder. Place one hand on your right ear to gently assist this motion. Stop when a stretch is felt in the muscles on the right side of your neck. Hold for a count of ten. Repeat the steps above in the opposite direction

Shoulders: Rotator Cuff, Deltoid Extension, Towel Stretch

Posterior Shoulder Stretch: Pretend you have an itch between your shoulder blades. Hold your left arm across your body and grab the back of your left elbow with your right hand. Pull the left elbow in as far as you can so that your left fingertips can reach your upper back. Repeat for the right shoulder.

Anterior Shoulder and Chest Stretch: Hold both hands behind your back, elbows extended. Now stick out your chest while you raise away from your body and hold. This stretches the lower back. Stand with your feet shoulder-width apart. Slowly bend forward at the waist and try to touch your toes. There is a huge degree of variation among people regarding how far they can go, so don't feel bad if you can't reach all the way to your toes. Remember not to bounce. If you have, you can sit on a bench and lean over to touch your toes. As with all stretches, only stretch to the point of "mild discomfort," not to the point of pain.

Front Arm

Biceps Stretch, Arm Extension, Wrist Extension: Position the arm from the hand to the inner elbow against a wall and turn the body away from it, exhaling slowly. This allows the stretching to occur in the biceps as well as the pectoral muscles. Hold this pose for 30 seconds and release slowly.

Arm Extension: Straighten the arms slowly and rotate the hands so they face down and lift the arms up. This can stretch the biceps, shoulders, and chest at the same time. Stand tall with good posture. Lift one arm forward then take it backward in a motion, keeping your spine long throughout. Perform this arm movement eight times before repeating with the other arm. Avoid the tendency to arch your spine while carrying out the movement. Breathe easily throughout.

Wrist Extension: Sit on the edge of a bench with a width of roughly 8-12 inches. Lean forward placing the forearms and elbows on the thighs. Move the wrists forward until they extend just beyond the patellae. Allow the wrists to flex toward the floor with upward movements, raise the 5-pound dumbbell by extending the wrists. Extend the wrists as far as possible without moving the elbows or forearms. Downward movements allow the wrists to slowly flex back to the starting position. Repeat 20-30 seconds.

Back Arm: Triceps Stretch, Arm Overhead Stretch

Triceps: Stand straight up with your legs shoulder-width apart. Bend your right arm at the elbow and touch the top of your shoulder blade with your fingers. Repeat on opposite arm.

Overhead Stretch: Reach over the top of your head with your left arm and grasp your right elbow. Gently pull with your left arm to increase the tension on the triceps muscle. Hold for 20-30 seconds. Repeat on your other arm.

Upper Back:

Trapezius Stretch: Grasp wrist or hand from behind and pull arm to opposite side. Tilt head away from lowered shoulder by positioning ear toward front of opposite shoulder. Hold stretch. Repeat to other side.

Lateral Bend: Grab a pair of 2-to 5-pound dumbbells and stand with your feet about four feet apart. Turn your left foot out 90 degrees. Raise your right arm straight up above your shoulder, palm facing in. Brace your abs and bend to the left, lowering the left dumbbell to your left ankle. Rise back up, keeping your right arm overhead. Do 10-15 repetitions then repeat on the other side. Do three sets, resting for up to 30 seconds between sets.

Prayer Stretch: Begin in a kneeling position with your hips pushed back and toes pointing straight out. Lower your chest toward your thighs. Extend your arms forward and overhead so they rest on floor, and curl mid back. Hold for 10 seconds. Without moving body position, walk hands to right and hold 10 seconds. Walk hands to left and hold 10 seconds, then walk hands to middle to return to start position. Repeat 3 times.

Chin-to-Chest Stretch: Gently bend your head forward while bringing your chin toward your chest. Stop when a stretch is felt in the back of your neck. Hold this position for 15 seconds. Return to starting position with your neck in midline position. Repeat above stretch 5 more times.

Lower Back: Knee-to-chest stretch, trunk twist, cat-and-camel stretch

Knee-to-Chest Stretch: Lie on your back with your knees and hips bent and the backs of your heels flat on the floor. Slowly pull one knee to your chest as far as you can.—You should feel a stretch in your lower back. Keep the opposite leg relaxed in a comfortable position. With your leg extended you can bend your knee if that feels better. Hold for 30 seconds and then repeat with the opposite leg.

Trunk Twist: Sit with your legs crossed. Reach your left hand toward your left foot and place your right hand at your side for support. Slowly twist your torso to your right. Switch your hands and twist to your left. Repeat left and right twists 5-10 times each. As with all stretches, only stretch to the point of "mild discomfort," not to the point of pain.

Cat-and-Camel Stretch: Lie on the floor in a hands and kneeling position. Place your knees shoulder width apart and align your hips so that your back and legs are at the right angle. Place your hands in front of you and make sure your shoulders are positioned so your back and arms are at the right angle. Your arms should be shoulder-width apart. Put your palms flat against the ground. Your arms should be engaged to support your weight, but don't lock your elbows. Start with the camel stretch: bend your back up toward the sky while rounding your neck and head toward your chest. Make sure your abdominal muscles are engaged and that your upper back is higher than your rounded shoulders. Your pelvis should naturally tilt toward your arms. Release in your lower back as you breathe in and out. Slowly move into the cat stretch as you arch your back toward the ground. Pull your shoulders back and bring your chin up toward the sky. As you slowly and fluidly arch your back, your pelvis should tilt out away from you, and your buttocks should rise into the air. Open your chest, engage your abdominals, and breathe. Repeat 4 times.

Buttocks:

Gluteus Stretch: Lie on your back with your right ankle crossed just below the left knee. Reach through with both hands to get a hold of the left knee. Gently pull the knee toward your chest and settle back, resting your head on the floor. Feel the stretch and hold for 10-30 seconds. If you are too stiff and cannot rest your head back on the floor, just hold the stretch for a shorter duration.

Oblique:

Oblique External and Internal Rotation Side to Side: Lie on your right side with your feet together. Place your right forearm on the ground so your elbow is under your shoulder and your left hand is on your hip. Raise your hips off the floor until you form a straight line with your head and your feet. Slowly lower your hips and repeat 12-15 times then switch sides. Do not strain your neck, keep it in line with your torso by concentrating on keeping the spine straight. As with all stretches, only stretch to the point of "mild discomfort," not to the point of pain.

Front Leg/Hip: Standing Lunge, Side Lunge, Quadriceps Stretch

Side-to-Side Leg Swings: a stretch for your hip adductors and abductors. Swing your leg from side to side while holding on to something. Move from the hips. Don't allow your torso to rotate. Keep your pelvis still, chest up and shoulder-blades back & down. Look forward. Point Your Feet Straight ahead. Lead with your heels to keep your feet pointing forward. This also improves ankle mobility. Take it slowly.

Split Squats: Assume a stance that's comfortable for you with your feet pointing forward. "Squat with both hands behind your head. Squeeze your glutes, increasing the stretch slowly prevent your lower back from arching. Squeeze the glute of your back leg on the way up. Push your knees out. Don't let your knees buckle in. Push from the heels, curl your toes if necessary push your knees out. Stand Tall! Look forward, keep your chest up and shoulder-blades back and down. Don't round your back, take it slowly.

Quadriceps Stretch: Stand up straight with your feet shoulder-width apart. Grab hold of a stationary object for balance. Lift your right leg off the ground, holding your ankle to your buttock with your knee pointed toward the floor, hips forward and level. (Don't let the right hip drop.) Engage your abdominal muscles to avoid arching your back. Feel the stretch in the front of your thigh hold the pose for 15-20 seconds. Repeat with the other leg.

Back Leg: Hamstring Stretch, Modified Hurdler Stretch

Hamstring Stretch: Sit on the floor with both legs out straight. Extend your arms and reach forward by bending at the waist as far as possible while keeping your knees straight. Hold this position for 10 seconds.

Modified Hurdler Stretch: Sit tall with your back straight, shoulders down, abs engaged, and legs extended like a V in front of you. Bend your left knee, placing the sole of your foot next to your inner right thigh. Rotate your torso to face your right leg. Bend forward from the waist, reaching your hands toward your toes. Imagine reaching your chin toward your toes in front of you (not toward your legs). Breathe deeply and hold for 10-30 seconds. Repeat on opposite side. As with all stretches, only to the point of "mild discomfort," not to the point of pain.

Lower Leg: Calf/Achilles, Ankle Inversion and Eversion Toe Extension.

Calf/Achilles Stretch: Stand facing a wall at about arm's length away. Stand with both feet facing straight ahead parallel not turned out. Put one foot on the wall at knee height. Press that heel toward the wall. Look down and see if the foot you are standing on is facing directly ahead. If not, make that standing foot straight, not turned out, not even a little. Do not lean toward the wall. Lift your chest until you are standing straight. Don't let your hip curl under or your standing knee or hip bend. Smile, relax your shoulders, and breathe. Hold a few seconds and switch legs.

Ankle Inversion and Eversion: Sit up straight with your back against a wall and your feet out in front of you with your knees straight. Slowly turn your left foot inward and hold this position for six seconds. Now turn your foot slowly outward and hold for another six seconds. Repeat this exercise on the opposite foot 3-set of 8 repetitions.

Toe Extension: Sit on a chair and place your ankle over the opposite knee. Grip toes and gently pull them back toward the knee while holding the ankle to prevent it from moving. Feel the stretch in the sole of the foot all the way to the heel. Hold the stretch for 30 seconds. Repeat three times for each foot.

As with all stretches, only stretch to the point of "mild discomfort," not to the point of pain.

You're done! You deserve it! Ten-minute stretch means better flexibility, which will help you stay limber with greater movement of all your body parts. So . . . S-t-r-e-t-c-h . . . S-t-r-e-t-c-h . . . S-t-r-e-t-c-h.

Notes

Notes

Notes

Notes

_____

_____

_____

_____

_____

_____

_____

_____

_____

_____

_____

_____

_____

_____

_____

_____

_____

_____

_____

_____

_____

_____

Notes

Notes

_____

_____

_____

_____

_____

_____

_____

_____

_____

_____

_____

_____

_____

_____

_____

_____

_____

_____

_____

_____

I have added these heart-healthy, low-caloric recipes as lagniappe, as we say in New Orleans. To encourage you on your journey to fitness through stretching, enjoy them and have fun with stretching.

Recipes

Cucumber Salad

1 1/2 Large, Thinly Sliced Cucumbers

1/2 cup. Plain Yogurt

1/2 tbsp. Sugar

1/2 tbsp. Vinegar

Salt and Pepper to taste

Mix well together yogurt, salt and pepper, sugar and vinegar.
fold in cucumber slices. Chill overnight.

Baked Fish

2lb. Salmon or Any Fish

1/2 cup. Olive Oil

3 tbsp. Garlic Powder

2 tbsp. Onion Powder

2 tbsp. Dry Parsley Flakes

1/2 tsp. Sugar

1 tbsp Worcestershire Sauce

1/2 cup. White Wine

1/4 tsp. Salt

1/4 tsp. Pepper

Season fish, on both sides with olive oil and salt and pepper place in open baking pan. Pour white wine over seasoned fish filets. Place in a 300-degree oven; cook for 10-12 minutes, basting occasionally. Serve with steamed vegetables

HEALTHY APPLE CAKE

2 cup. Diced Apples

1 cup. Sugar

1/3 cup. Corn Oil

1/2 tsp. Vanilla

2 Beaten Egg Whites

1 1/2 cup. White Flour

1 tsp. Baking Powder

1 tsp. Soda

1 tsp. Cinnamon

1/2 cup. Raisins

Combine apples and sugar and let it stand 10 minutes. Blend oil, vanilla, and egg with the apples. Then combine the dry mix and mix well. stir in raisins. Pour into greased 8-inch square pan. Bake at 350 degrees for 45 minutes.

Feel Great, Look Great